Strength Training Over 40

The Ultimate Workout Plan

Gabriel Montgomery

Copyright © 2022 by Gabriel Montgomery

All rights reserved.

No portion of this book may be reproduced in any form without written permission from the publisher or author, except as permitted by U.S. copyright law.

Contents

1. Reps and Sets — 1
2. The Ultimate Workout Plan — 21
3. Healing — 40
4. Essential Nutrients — 53
5. Maintaining Consistency — 76
6. FAQs — 90

Chapter 1

Reps and Sets

A set of exercises is a collection of reps carried out in a certain order. You've finished one set of 8 repetitions, for instance, if you take up a kettlebell, do 8 military presses with it, and then put it back. You would have finished two sets of eight repetitions if you took a break and then repeated the exercise.

Perform one set of each exercise if you are just beginning a strength training regimen. According to research, beginners to strength training can achieve the same results with one set of each exercise as they would with three sets.

This is due to the fact that muscles respond more quickly to a resistance workout in untrained people since their beginning strength is always low. There's space for improvement here. Additionally, concentrating on doing 1 set of each exercise at the beginning can help you learn the movements and prevent injuries.

The good news is that this noticeable and immediate improvement encourages you to keep exercising. However, strength increases seem to plateau after three to four months. To get the desired muscular improvement, you must then raise the number of sets each exercise to three to five.

On the other hand, repetition or reps refer to the quantity of times you carry out a certain strength-training exercise in a set. The ideal range for reps each set is between 6 and 12. The lower end of this spectrum focuses more on strength and power, while the upper end is more concerned with muscle endurance.

Changing the number of reps completed per set, the weight or load being lifted, the number of sets, the time under stress, or the pace at which you perform the exercise can all have an impact on how your muscles react.

The most crucial thing to understand about repetitions per set is that, depending on whether your main objective for strength training is to increase muscle endurance or strength and power, you want to hit physical failure within the 6–12 range or any other range of your choice.

If gaining power and strength is your main objective, you should only execute exercises for 1–6 reps; after that, you have reached muscle failure and cannot complete any more reps. If you are unable to complete one rep, the weight is too heavy for you. Additionally, if you are able to complete more than 6 repetitions, the weight is too light for you to use for building strength and power.

You should be able to complete 12 or more reps if building muscle endurance is your main objective. If you are unable to complete the 12th rep, the weight is too heavy for your muscles to lift.

In conclusion, the quantity of sets completed in an exercise varies based on your training objectives. The following list of suggested sets is provided by the National Strength and Conditioning Association (NSCA) (Kamb, 2021):

You must complete 2-3 sets of 12 to 20+ reps if you want to develop muscle endurance.

You must execute 3-6 sets of 6–12 reps if you want to develop muscular hypertrophy.

You should execute 2–6 sets of no more than 6 repetitions if your training objective is to increase muscle strength.

Remember that these ranges are ideal for developing strength or muscle. That does not imply that if you complete 4 sets, you will only increase your strength but not your muscle mass, and that if you perform 10 reps, you will only increase your muscle mass but not your strength.

According to certain research, you can even build the same muscles by doing numerous reps with light weights till failure. I favor doing it the other way around, with higher weights and less repetitions. Performing 3x10 reps as an example rather than 3x30. This allows for time savings and a sharper focus on appropriate body positioning and movement techniques.

In light of the aforementioned recommendations, I advise executing three sets of 6–12 reps in order to gain the advantages of both muscle and strength development. Remember to choose a weight that is sufficiently difficult. When you can complete more than 12 repetitions, it's time to increase the weight or employ other techniques of progression. If you are unable to complete 6 repetitions, the weight is too heavy (I will introduce them to you further in this chapter). Therefore, if you are able to execute more reps than are necessary to reach a particular objective, it is time to increase the weight in order to advance in your workout.

I advise getting a weight that you can lift no more than six times before doing anything else. If you are not a complete beginner, it can take you around a year before you can perform more than 12 repetitions with this weight before you need to replace it. Similar to this, you might try other progression strategies to advance in your workouts before raising the weight.

Repeating Rate

Repetition speed is the rate at which you raise and drop the weight during each repetition (weight, in this case, includes body weight too, and lift also refers to the upward movement of your weight regardless of the direction your body moves). It is simply the amount of time needed to complete each iteration.

The duration under strain increases as a rep or set is taken longer to finish. Slow down the movement if an exercise gets so simple that you can perform more repetitions than is advised. Spend more time concentrating when you exercise your muscles completely. This increases the strength, endurance, and growth of your muscles by making them work harder.

Reduce your tempo to extend your time under tension during your workout. A pace of 1:1:1 would suggest that you would take one second to lower your body, one second to pause in the squat position, and one second to stand up and return to the starting position when performing the kettlebell goblet squat.

If you have no trouble doing it, try slowing down the movement to a pace of 2:1:2, 3:1:3, and so on. Increase the weight you're using when you can comfortably finish the movements at a 5:1:5 speed.

Although your preferred repeat speed will influence it to some extent, it is essential to accomplish all of your workout repetitions under control. When we say something is "under control," we typically mean that it is being repeated quickly without requiring momentum or inertia (this is not the case for kettlebell swing). Your body is put under more strain when your muscles are under more control, which also lowers your risk of injury.

The stop test is one of the best methods for evaluating your repetition speed. During a repetition, try halting the exercise at any point along the movement's range. You are utilizing the proper repetition speed if you can stop. To find out if you are completing your repetitions at the right pace throughout your workouts, use this test.

Exercise Weight/Load

The first safety consideration for anyone doing strength training is always choosing a suitable exercise resistance or load. Making ensuring that your starting weight is not too heavy is crucial. The weight you lift or the amount of resistance you apply to an exercise set greatly influences how many repetitions you accomplish.

If building muscle strength is your primary objective, you should choose a weight that will allow you to perform 1-6 repetitions without discomfort. When you can complete more repetitions with the same loads while still exercising with these weights, raise or modify the resistance by applying the overload principle.

Rest Time Between Exercises and Sets

A rest period is the interval between sets during which you rest to give your muscles a chance to heal. The typical rest interval between sets is between 30 and 2 minutes (Rogers, 2020). Consequently, give your muscles 1-2 minutes to rest between sets when you execute two or more sets of the same exercise. This amount of time is necessary to recuperate your muscles and replenish the majority of the energy consumed during the workouts.

You must also give your muscles a brief break in between sets of exercises in order to lessen the overall impact of tiredness on succeeding muscular efforts. The typical amount of time needed to recover between exercises is 1-2 minutes.

For various training objectives, the rest period between exercise sets typically falls within the following ranges:

The rest period between sets should be between two and five minutes if you want to increase muscle strength.

The rest period between sets during an activity should be between 30 and 60 seconds if you want to build muscle endurance.

The rest period between workout sets should be between 30 and 90 seconds if your training objective is muscular growth.

After finishing your activity, you can take a little break to get your breathing back to normal before moving on to the next. I work in that field. I don't always time myself to make sure I take exactly 1-2 minutes to relax in between workouts.

Breathing Technique

Regardless of the kind and degree of the workout you are doing, never hold your breath while strength training. Holding your breath might increase inside pressure, which could prevent blood from flowing freely. This could cause symptoms like dizziness and high blood pressure reactions, which would interfere with your training. Breathe consistently during your training sessions to avoid these negative consequences.

Always inhale during the simpler lowering or return phase of each repetition and exhale during the most challenging phase of the repetition (difficult lifting, pushing, or pulling), also known as the sticking point. This keeps a better internal pressure response in place. You are encouraged to breathe properly during each repetition of your complete workout because it is a necessary component of safe strength training exercises.

Body Shape

The way your body is positioned as you exercise matters more than the amount of weight you use or the number of sets and reps you do. During workouts, focusing on form might help you perform better and build muscle.

Here are a few advantages of exercising with proper form:

It aids in avoiding accidents. You can prevent problems related to flexibility and weight by exercising with good technique. Your muscles are put under extra stress when you lift weights, whether it be your own body weight, free weight, or anything else. Additionally, because every component of your body is interconnected, if one is out of balance, the others will also malfunction. For instance, if you squat improperly, your spine could get hurt.

It lessens the amount of energy lost during activity. You have to exert more effort and extra energy when executing the workouts when you are exercising with poor form. You might expend significantly less energy to do the same activity if you exercise with good body form. Your workout also becomes effortless and fun! No bending over.

It increases the efficiency and efficacy of workouts. You can have a useful workout experience when you use proper form while performing an exercise. You can experience total extension and contraction of muscles as a result of being able to move your joints and muscles through their full range of motion, which leads to greater results.

Even though the terms "posture" and "form" may seem straightforward and commonplace, most people do not carry out their workouts with the right bodily form. But you must be aware that using good form is crucial to reaching your fitness objectives. By lowering muscle stresses, it makes exercising pain-free for you. Additionally, it enables you to exercise the targeted muscles properly.

Motion Range

How far your joints can move with each rep is referred to as your range of motion. In other words, it relates to your joints' capacity to carry out the whole range of motions you do while exercising. The majority of specialists advise exercising while using all of your joints' ranges of motion. I also advise it. According to studies, building full-range muscular strength requires exercising your body in all directions.

When you exercise over your entire range of motion, your muscles will fully stretch and fully contract. In other words, when the target muscle group stretches all the way, the opposing muscle group contracts all the way, and vice versa.

Your biceps and triceps serve as a good illustration; when your elbow joint moves through its full range of motion, your biceps fully stretch and your triceps fully contract. Naturally, you shouldn't go beyond your joints' natural range of motion or experience any discomfort when moving. Eliminate any exercise that makes your joints hurt or uncomfortable, and make sure you only exercise within a range of motion that is pain-free.

The following advantages come from exercising with a wide range of motion:

Enhances joint flexibility. Your joint flexibility will increase by working through the entire range of motion during your activities. When it comes to strengthening your body, flexibility is crucial since it supports good posture and weight-lifting techniques. Consequently, you must carry out your exercise through its entire range of motion if you want your workout to be more effective and efficient.

allows you to workout more and with less effort. A broad range of joint motion during exercise enables you to complete more difficult workouts while using less energy. According to studies, persons who exercise their muscles through their full range of motion build up their muscle strength, which enables them to lift bigger objects without exerting too much effort.

Exercise Progression

Most of us want to develop in our workouts. But other people always stick to what feels more natural to them, which is doing the same number of reps or sets with the same amount of weight. The main training principle, the progressive overload principle, is in tension with this.

According to the progressive overload concept, you must gradually raise your muscle's working load in order to confront your body and muscles with fresh training stimuli if you want to continue increasing strength and muscle mass or making other exercise-related progress.

Keep in mind that not all exercises advance at the same rate. And once more, avoid packing on the pounds quickly or accelerating your progress by sacrificing form. Instead, you will harm your body even more.

Even while most people follow this rule when moving from one workout to another, many do it incorrectly. It is not a question of your lifting capacity. The most important factor is whether you can perform it correctly.

Lifting lesser weights in full-range reps will help you avoid injuries and achieve better results than doing half-assed reps with heavy weights. Not that bigger loads and half-reps are terrible. No. What I'm trying to say is that it's right and safer to establish your form with the full range version first.

Use a larger load while maintaining the same reps, sets, rest intervals, and tempo to increase your weight. You may raise 52.5 pounds the following time you do the same exercise, for instance, if you are presently lifting 50 pounds. According to studies, increasing your weight load by as low as 2.5 pounds at each stage of your training progression is both safe and beneficial. However, using a single dumbbell or kettlebell makes that less straightforward, so I favor other development techniques.

Other Methods of Progress

I already explained how you can speed up your progress by using heavier weights or longer periods of strain. You can use various progression techniques to make sure you're continually moving forward with your fitness objectives:

Upping the number of sets. Add one set while keeping the weight and rest duration constant to advance your sets. For instance, if you are performing an activity with 50 lbs for 3 sets of 10 reps, you can perform the exercise with 4 sets of 10 reps the following time.

Gain more reps. Add one more rep to each set while keeping the weight and rest duration the same to advance your reps. For instance, the next time you perform the same workout, consider performing three sets of six repetitions with the same weight if you are now lifting 50 lbs for three sets of five.

shortening your sleep duration. Maintain the weight and reps/sets while reducing the rest between sets. The workout becomes more difficult as a result. For instance, if you typically take two minutes off between sets of a certain exercise, try cutting it down to one minute and thirty seconds while still using the same weight and executing the same amount of sets and reps.

What counts most when strength training is how we perform our exercises. You must take into account all the previously mentioned variables if you want your workout to be both physically and mentally beneficial. The exercises presented should be correctly completed in order to develop the muscle memory and pathway needed for long-term outcomes. You can do this by simply adhering to the tips and recommendations offered in this book.

Now that you have a practical grasp and respect of these training principles, I think you're ready to follow the straightforward workout plan I've created for you in the following chapter. Remember that to continue progressing in your workouts, you must maintain the proper training intensity, which is influenced by the aforementioned concepts.

Main Points

Be mindful to exercise with good form and posture. Make sure your joints can move completely when you are lifting weights.

Breathing should never be held during exercising. It is best to inhale during the simpler lowering or return portion of each repetition and exhale during the most challenging aspect of the repetition (difficult lifting, pushing, or pulling).

Between sets and exercises, take 1-2 minutes to rest to give your muscles a chance to recuperate.

To get the most out of your exercises, perform three sets of 6–12 repetitions of each exercise.

You will get the best results with the least amount of effort if you aim to work out twice a week.

Chapter 2

The Ultimate Workout Plan

What factors influence a weightlifting program's success? Your diligence and commitment.

Craig Everett

I hope this book has been educational up to this point and that you have gained some ideas, thoughts, or views to help you begin your strength training adventure. Exercises do not become workouts unless they are planned and organized into a program, and a workout program cannot assist you in successfully achieving your training objectives unless it is user-friendly, creative, and efficient.

I've done just that in this chapter. Let's first understand something about muscle preparation prior to a workout and cool down following a workout before we begin the training program. You probably want to know what supersets are and why we're using them in our program because we're also going to execute our workouts in them.

Both pre- and post-workout

It can be tempting to forgo a warm-up at times, especially if you are pressed for time or just eager to get started with your workout. The physiological and psychological advantages of warming up before participating in vigorous physical activity are, nevertheless, extremely substantial.

One of the demanding exercises that puts a lot of strain on your musculoskeletal system is strength training. As a result, it is crucial to warm up before beginning a strength exercise. Jumping rope, jogging while stationary, and brisk walking are all excellent strategies to quickly warm up before your workout. You should only need 2 to 5 minutes to complete these warm-up activities.

advantages of pre-warming

reduces the chance of harm. The last thing you should experience after consistently exercising is sprains, strains, or other types of ailments. Warming up your muscles increases their suppleness, which lowers your risk of injury or overheating while exercising.

mentally gets you ready for what's coming. It can be quite simple to lose motivation and stop working out when things get tough. You are less likely to do this, though, if you warm up before the workout. This is due to the fact that when you warm up, your brain concentrates on your body and the exercise; this focus carries over into your training session and serves to remind you of your fitness objectives.

improves adaptability. Your muscles will be more mobile and simpler to control as a result of warm-up exercises.

increases oxygen and blood flow. A 5-minute warm-up that includes a simple exercise like jogging while stationary helps to open blood vessels and improve blood flow to your skeletal muscles. This aids in providing your muscles with the necessary amount of oxygen as you exercise, eliminating what is frequently referred to as "oxygen debt."

After your workout, cooling down is just as crucial as warming up. The fundamental goal of cooling down is to gradually return your blood pressure and heart rate to normal following activity. In a sense, this time is the warm-up in reverse.

Your heart has been beating faster and harder than usual throughout the entire workout, so it's crucial to gradually return to normal rather than stopping suddenly.

For older people, the cool-down is especially crucial because it prevents the buildup of blood and other bodily fluids in the lower legs, which could result in unfavorable changes in blood pressure and cardiovascular issues.

Stretching exercises after a 5- to 10-minute cool-down exercise like brisk walking help the body return to normal blood flow and heart rate more easily.

The necessity of cooling off

It promotes muscle healing. Following a vigorous workout, lactate builds up in the blood, making it acidic. This causes your musculoskeletal system to accumulate lactic acid. It takes time for your body to rid itself of the lactic acid. Exercises for cooling down thereby improve the process of lactic acid release and removal, accelerating muscle repair.

reduces DOMS (Delayed Onset Muscle Soreness). Muscle aches and pains are common after an exercise, but having a lot of DOMS can be uncomfortable and keep you from doing out again. According to research, cooling down after an exercise helps reduce extreme muscle soreness, which makes you feel more at ease and prepared for the next activity.

Stretching

It is a good idea to stretch. Even if you don't exercise frequently, stretching should still be a part of your daily routine. It maintains the flexibility and range of motion of your muscles. The American College of Sports Medicine advises stretching your major muscle groups for 60 seconds apiece, at least twice a week (Collins, 2012).

Should you warm up by stretching?

Static stretching shouldn't be done prior to exercise. There is no evidence that static stretching before exercise can enhance performance or assist prevent injury or reduce muscular soreness after exercise. In fact, studies suggest that static stretching alone prior to exercise might reduce your muscular strength and power and deteriorate your performance (Simic, 2013).

You should instead warm up by performing vigorous stretches.

After working out, should you stretch?

The ideal moment to stretch is right now. After exercising, static stretching can help you recuperate, chill down, and get ready for the next workout. Stretching now will assist increase blood flow, which will help transport nutrients and oxygen to the sore muscles, promoting healing and rejuvenation. Additionally, it aids in heart rate lowering and nervous system relaxation.

How to safely stretch

If you must stretch before working out, make sure your muscles are not fully cold before you begin. Before stretching your muscles, you should engage in some warm-up exercises to help your muscles create heat. This can be accomplished by shaking various body parts, such as your hands, arms, and legs.

Hold the stretch for at least 30 seconds if it is static, which is typically done after a workout. Allow your body enough time to process the extension. Your tissues will be lot safer with this. Try to exert more pressure while on the verge. You shouldn't experience any pain while stretching. If you do, stop immediately since you are not performing the action properly. Give it some thought and do it right.

Supersets

Simply said, this involves doing two separate workouts back-to-back with little to no break in between.

advantages of supersets

They reduce waiting time. When you're pressed for time, supersets are fantastic. Your workout will be shorter but more fruitful if you do two separate exercises with no or little rest in between. I can finish my whole-body workout in about 30 minutes by using supersets.

heightened intensity With the aid of supersets, you may accomplish more in less time, maximizing the benefits of your exercise regimen.

enhances muscular endurance Supersets assist in preparing your muscles to work out for longer amounts of time. This makes you stronger and enables you to continue working out for longer.

They aid in increasing calorie burn. Supersets have been shown in numerous studies to increase calorie burn both during and after exercise.

improving active rest. By doing supersets, you work one muscle while the opposing one relaxes. This maximizes fat burning and muscular building.

The Initiative

The best compound exercises, the actual core muscle-building motions that were described in Chapter 4, are one of the most crucial things you need to be performing when it comes to muscle-building training. You must strengthen those as well.

For you to make improvement, performing those exercises consistently while following a tried-and-true program is especially important if you're over 40 or 50.

Once we've mastered the complex actions, we must additionally comprehend the ideal frequency at which to practice. There are many various techniques to train for muscle growth, and frequency essentially refers to how frequently we hit a muscle region. Each of them has advantages of its own.

The majority of the time, these bodybuilding publications will advise you to really divide up your training schedule: for example, just work on your chest on Monday, your back on Tuesday, your shoulders on Wednesday, your legs on Thursday, and your arms on Friday. These split routines are really specialized, and it turns out that with this type of training, you essentially just do a ton of chest sets on Monday before skipping chest for another five to seven days. For the majority of us, that is not the best approach to train. I advise you to train more frequently but with fewer sets per session. That implies you should train your chest two to three times per week, with enough recuperation in between sessions, rather than performing a lot of sets on Monday.

Every time you work out a muscle, a few days after the workout, you experience a protein synthesis muscle-building stimulus. However, this stimulus only lasts for a few days, and you must work out again to experience it. Not much more protein synthesis occurs when we slam our chest with 20 sets than when we only perform a few challenging sets. By performing 20 sets for each muscle group, we merely add more recovery time, which prolongs the soreness. After that, we won't be able to train for a further five to seven days.

As we grow into our 40s and 50s, it's even more optimal to spread out that volume even more with 2 to 3 full body workouts, where you're performing all the finest compound exercises dispersed throughout the week. This is because we perform the ideal amount of sets and allow ample time for recovery. The body is hit more frequently, which keeps the stimulation for muscular growth consistent. So, choosing the correct routines and volume is crucial for achieving your training goals.

I have incorporated workouts that are quite effective on their own in the regimen below. This program makes the most of this effectiveness while requiring the least amount of work, giving you fantastic results.

Practical Advice

Perform push-ups and goblet squats without stopping (superset #1). After performing these two movements once, take a quick break (about a minute) before performing superset #1. Rest for a few minutes before moving on to supersets #2, #3, and #4 after performing superset #1 a total of three times. I advise you to complete 6–12 repetitions of each exercise.

Due to their simplicity, ability to target a variety of muscle groups, and effectiveness as a warm-up exercise, push-ups and squats are where I've started. Since swing is the riskiest exercise for beginners and I prefer to perform it after three supersets, you should be adequately warmed up. Supersets will help you complete your workout more quickly, but you can also perform standard sets in their place. In these, you perform one exercise for three sets with a 1-2 minute break between each set, and only then move on to the next exercise. Chapter 4 discussed these and all other fundamental exercises. If you need to substitute any of my suggested workouts, you can discover all the alternate exercises there.

However, it's crucial to understand that there are a variety of methods to organize your training regimen; the framework I've provided here is not fixed. It can be adjusted and modified according to your training objectives. This can, however, be a terrific and sustainable training strategy for you, as it is for me, if you want to achieve tremendous results with the least bit of effort.

Try to include exercises that make use of the barbell, pull-up bar, or parallel bars if you have access to them throughout your workout. When I have access to this equipment, I love to use it to execute exercises like pull-ups in place of rows and incline bench presses in place of push-ups. But if you are unable to access this equipment, don't be puzzled. The most crucial thing is to do out the aforementioned compound workouts using any available equipment, or even without.

Both the dumbbell and kettlebell are reliable tools for enhancing one's level of fitness. You can also use a pair of dumbbells to accomplish similar complex movements:

Exercise Program Using Dumbbells

Dumbbell Swing Hinge (or Dumbbell Deadlift)

Pull: Dumbbell Row with One Arm (or Two-Arm Dumbbell Row)

Dumbbell Bench Press: Push-ups (or Incline Dumbbell Bench Press)

Squat with a dumbbell (or Dumbbell Lunges)

Seated dumbbell press: Vertical Press (or Standing Dumbbell Press)

Center: Leg lift (or Crunch, Plank)

A workout regimen with free weights that is above intermediate will likely be the best fit for you if you have some resistance training experience or are returning to it after a break.

Can novices use dumbbells and kettlebells for exercise?

Absolutely, yes. Beginners can use free weights without difficulty, but it's important to emphasize that during the first few exercises, form should come before focus. I advise beginning with beginner workout routines using lighter weights, resistance bands, or only bodyweight exercises if you are very new to exercise, recovering from an injury, prefer low-intensity strength training, have physical limitations that could impair movement patterns, or any of these situations apply to you.

Everyone wishing to simply tone their muscles, maintain their strength, and maintain daily health from the comfort of home or while traveling may benefit from resistance band or bodyweight exercises.

These exercises are a priceless resource for bodybuilders looking for a hard training session when the gym is out of their price range as well as elders looking to increase their strength and body composition without having to own a gym.

Not everyone who desires to get stronger and more healthy can or wants to visit a gym. They might not have the time. They could choose to work up a sweat in the privacy of their own home because the cost of a gym membership is out of their budget or because they don't feel at ease in a gym setting. And if this applies to you, a bodyweight exercise program is a perfect choice:

Exercise using Bodyweight: Hip Raise (or Standing Back Extensions)

Bodyweight Row: Pull (or Doorway rows)

Push-ups on the knees (or Wall, Incline, Decline Pushups)

Bodyweight Squats (or Chair, Box squats, Bodyweight Lunge)

Push-up variation: the vertical press (or Incline pike push-up)

Leg Lift While Lying (or Crunch, Plank)

Exercise with resistance bands: Deadlift with Resistance Band

Resistance-band rows, pull

a resistance band for pushups Push-ups

Squats using resistance bands

Press vertically while using a resistance band.

Leg Lift While Lying (or Crunch, Plank)

Advanced exercises with a barbell will probably suit you best if you're stronger as you go along and feel like you need something harder to challenge your muscle strength, or if you've had a lot of experience with bodyweight training or weightlifting and you're looking for more challenging weights and workouts.

Although barbell exercises are not for everyone, many people think that barbell exercises make up the bulk of the best strength training regimens since they enable you to build muscle and strength more quickly than any other type of exercise. After several years of adequate training, this may not be enough to produce progressive overload on movements like the squat, deadlift, bench press, and dumbbell row, even if it is enough to progress on most exercises using bodyweight or any equipment. The best barbell exercises to increase strength and muscle growth are the following if you are an experienced lifter and wish or are able to visit a gym:

Hinge: Barbell Workout Routine Barbell Deadlift

Barbell Bent Over Row: Pull (or Pull-Up)

Barbell Bench Press: Push-ups (or Incline Barbell Bench Press)

Squat: Back Squat with a Bar (or Barbell Front Squat)

Barbell Overhead Press: Vertical Press (or Military Press)

Basic: Raise a hanging leg (or Incline Crunch, Plank)

Main Points

Pre-warm up before beginning any exercise.

Supersets are a fantastic time-saving strategy.

Concentrate on compound movements rather than specific exercises or pieces of equipment.

Your workouts will become even more efficient and enjoyable if you occasionally switch up the exercises or equipment you use.

Chapter 3

Healing

Unknown "If you're not asking for rest, you're not training your best"

For a healthy, strong physique and optimum physical fitness, regular exercise is essential. You must give your muscles enough time to recuperate, though, if you want to get the most out of your regular workouts and achieve your ideal body shape without getting hurt.

Even if they go above and beyond by increasing the amount of reps/sets and utilizing proper lifting techniques, some people who workout in gyms or at home with high-end gym equipment and free weights still don't see the results of their labors.

I have no doubt that you have come across such individuals, and they may have in some way discouraged you. Don't let them stop you from exercising. Not the workouts, the issue. Failure to give your muscles enough time to recuperate is likely the culprit here.

The majority of individuals are mistaken about how strength training contributes to the development of muscular mass and strength in the body. They believe that exercise causes muscles to grow. Because of this, many people frequently ignore the idea of a recovery period. You must realize that growing muscles takes place during recovery time, not during the actual workout period. After the workout, that is.

The health of your muscles may suffer long-term consequences if you ignore the healing regimen. In this chapter, I'll go through the idea of recuperation, how it might benefit our bodies after exercise, and how to do it. Read on!

Muscle Recovery: What Is It?

The energy that is stored in your muscles is used up during a strength training activity, which causes your muscles to get fatigued and lose strength. More energy is produced and stored in your muscles throughout the recovery period. More than just giving your muscles enough time to cease hurting is involved in muscle recovery. I'll teach you strategies to hasten your recovery later in this chapter.

Recovery of muscles is crucial.

Think again if you believe that skipping a day of exercise will always set you back. The fact is, you must give your body enough time to recover from your previous workout after working out before working out again.

Most people who train frequently tend to overlook the notion that exercise is stress. Yes it is. But wait..., did this statement confuse you? Did you just read somewhere in the previous chapters that exercises reduce stress? Don't get confused. This is not the same type of stress I am talking about. This is good stress. Exercise stresses your muscles which provides long-lasting benefits in the end.

Any intense exercise creates fatigue, micro-traumas, and tears in your muscles. Muscle soreness and pain are the most common symptoms of this effect. If you don't allow your muscles to heal and recover from this damage, it can prevent your muscles' ability to replenish their glycogen stores.

After exercise, lactic acid accumulates within your body cells. There is scientific evidence that lactic acid impairs the electrical stimulus required for muscle contraction when it builds up in your muscles. It also impairs your body's ability to generate ATP which is an essential molecule that plays a big role in repeated muscle contraction.

None of the above sounds beneficial, right? It is until you factor in the recovery period that's when you will enjoy the fruits of your workout efforts. For these micro-traumas and tears to repair, we need to create a healing environment for them. It is through recovery that your body will get rid of lactic acid from your muscles and restore its capacity to produce ATP.

What happens if you don't recover?

For beginners, you won't see good results from your workout. Overworking your muscles without giving them enough time to recover doesn't yield the desired fitness outcome.

Lack of sleep during the night is another sign of inadequate recovery after exercise. Overtraining makes it hard for your body to differentiate fatigue from exercise with other stressors. As a result, your body enters into a chronic dominant state of fight-or-flight, making you too wired to sleep.

Another indication that you're not having enough recovery time from your exercise is cravings for sweet or salty foods. During exercise, most of us sweat a lot, in the process, we lose electrolytes. This creates electrolyte imbalance in your body making you crave such foods. Research has also associated a lack of muscle recovery with hormonal upset and impaired immune function.

Ways in Which Our Muscles Recover

Stretching, rest, nutrition, hydration, sleep, and massage are the six elements of muscle recovery. Let's take a closer look at each element in detail.

1. Stretching

Stretching is an important aspect of exercise, that's why it is recommended that you include it in your workout routine. But, many people tend to neglect it. Dynamic stretching before a workout keeps your body open giving your muscles space and flexibility to complete the moves safely and through a full range of motion. This helps reduce the risks of injury, muscle soreness, and tears. On the other hand, stretching after a workout helps heal your muscles and reduce DOMS. (For more information on the benefits of stretching, refer to chapter 6 of this book.)

2. Rest Days

If you are following a workout program, you will always hear people remind you about your workout days and how you need to exercise regularly. But you will never hear anyone talk about rest. Rest days are as important as workout days.

To achieve your training goals, you must include rest days in your workout routine and adhere to them. They help your body repair and recover faster. As discussed earlier, the process of muscle building takes 2-4 days. And while most experts recommend fullbody strength training for 2-3 nonconsecutive days per week, this may vary from person to person. The good news is that there is a way your body communicates when it needs rest.

Signs that you need Rest

If you notice any of the following signs, know that your body needs rest and it will help if you plan for a rest day:

Decreased performance. If you stop seeing progress, or you start having difficulties in carrying out your exercises, take a rest day.

Lack of sleep. If you can't sleep for at least 7-8 hours every night, take some rest from your workout.

Sore muscles. Although it is quite common and normal to feel sore after your workout, it shouldn't go for a prolonged period. If the soreness is persistent, you need to take action. It is a sign that your muscles are yet to recover from the previous workouts and they need some time to do so.

Pain. Consistent pain in your muscles and joints might be a sign of injuries from overuse.

Muscle fatigue. You need to rest if you feel extremely exhausted.

3. Nutrition

Both exercise and diet contribute in equal measure to the fitness equation. Consuming protein after working out is important since it aids in refueling and muscle rehabilitation. You are aware by this point that regular exercise causes your muscles to experience microtrauma and rips. You will want amino acids in order to rebuild and repair these muscles. This means that in order to help provide the amino acid to your muscles, you will need to consume protein.

You already know that your body burns glycogen during exercise, and that by the time you're done, your glycogen reserves will be low. You must eat some carbohydrates as well in order to refill your glycogen reserves. Continue reading because I will cover nutrition and exercise in greater detail in the following chapter.

4. Water intake

Your body loses water and electrolytes through perspiration when you exercise. Dehydration from this could impair your performance. To keep your body properly hydrated, it is essential that you consume lots of water prior to, during, and after the workout.

The normal advice is to make sure you consume at least 8 glasses, or 2 liters, of water each day. Electrolyte water can be a wonderful alternative since aside keeping your body hydrated, it also supplies your body with critical electrolytes like calcium, potassium, and magnesium which also play a part in muscle rehabilitation.

5. Sleep

Rapid Eye Movement (REM) and Non-Rapid Eye Movement (NREM) are the two main phases of sleep (Non-REM). You must comprehend what transpires during these two sleep phases if you want to comprehend how sleep affects muscle healing. Sleep with rapid eye movement (REM)

About 25% of your entire sleep time is spent in this sleep stage. All through the night, it happens in cycles that last roughly 1.5 to 2 hours. The latter half of your sleep is dominated by REM sleep. It gives your brain the fuel it needs to function during the day. Your mind is also restored by it.

REM-Free Sleep

The most crucial stage of muscle rehabilitation is this one. It is the location of deep sleep. It is referred to as the slowwave or deep sleep phase for this reason.

It makes up roughly 40% of your overall sleep. Your breathing grows slower and deeper during this phase, and your blood pressure drops.

Because it is resting, there aren't many activity happening in your brain right now. The blood flow to your muscles rises as a result, providing them with more oxygen and nourishment. Faster healing and muscle growth are enhanced by this.

The release of growth hormones is a crucial event that takes place during this sleep stage. Your pituitary glands release a burst of growth hormones as your body enters this phase, promoting muscle recovery and tissue growth. The secretion of growth hormones can suddenly fall if you don't get enough sleep at night.

According to research, a lack of growth hormones is linked to decreased exercise tolerance and a loss of muscle mass.

In conclusion, growth hormone secretion and protein synthesis are two ways that sleep improves muscle rehabilitation. It is crucial to get at least 7-8 hours of sleep per night if you want to gain muscle mass and recover from prior workouts more quickly.

Massage 6.

After exercise, give your muscles a massage. The lactic acids that accumulate in the exercised muscles are reduced by massaging the areas. This facilitates a quicker recovery.

7. Sauna

Saunas offer a number of health advantages in addition to being a soothing method to wind down after exercise. Blood arteries expand when exposed to high temperatures, which improves circulation and decreases blood pressure.

Saunas are used by certain sportsmen to improve their stamina and performance. Saunas might be useful for enhancing your strength and power as well. Your comfort level will determine how long you spend in the sauna, but generally speaking, for most healthy adults, 15 minutes is a reasonable time limit.

Main Points

It is crucial to get enough rest after working out since the muscles that have been stressed require time to recover and regenerate. Limit your muscular use. Spend some time sleeping well. Make sure you get 7-8 hours of sleep each night.

To keep your body hydrated and replenish the electrolytes lost through perspiration during exercise, drink plenty of water, especially one that contains electrolytes. The usual advice is to drink at least 8 glasses every day.

Chapter 4

Essential Nutrients

We would have discovered the most secure path to health if we could provide each individual with the ideal quantity of nutrition and activity, neither too little nor too much.

— Hippocrates

Nutrition and exercise go hand in hand. One cannot ever be discussed without the other. If you want to have a healthy, strong, and attractive figure, you must exercise and follow a balanced diet.

Eating healthy doesn't necessarily mean sticking to bland things like salads. It shouldn't feel more like self-denial than self-improvement when you're on a diet.

I'm trying to imply that you can create a healthy diet plan with the things you enjoy. You don't have to give up your favorite foods because of a "clean eating" compulsion.

Depending on your fitness objective, you'll decide which diet to follow. Less calories must be consumed if you want to lose weight, whereas more calories must be consumed if you want to build weight and muscle mass.

It's simply basic biology, but what I've discovered over the years is that you don't have to starve yourself in order to lose weight, and you also don't have to stuff yourself silly whenever you get the chance in order to gain weight or muscle mass. Both of these viewpoints are extremely harmful and potentially fatal, as anyone with a clear head would realize.

The first thing you need to understand is that everyone has a unique body type and metabolic system. A diet that is most effective for one individual might not be for you. As a result, while trying to establish a new eating regimen, base it on your existing habits.

For instance, if you regularly eat four meals a day and are trying to lose weight, reduce that number to three.

Therefore, when we boil everything down, it really just comes down to regulated, scheduled eating in moderation. Regardless of your training objectives, you must consume as few processed and sugary "foods" as feasible.

What is the most crucial aspect of fitness, then, is a topic of discussion. Eating right or exercising? Others claim that nutrition and other factors are more significant than exercise, while some claim that exercise is the most important element. Some continue to assert that one is 40% and the other is 60%. In case you weren't aware, diet is crucial.

Is my voice crazy? You must be thinking how much of an impact exercise has. Exercise also counts as 100%.

Although there are additional elements, these two are the most important. Does that sound strange? I am aware of your confusion on the overall percentage.

Yes, it can increase by up to 1,000%. The key takeaway is that a superb body's components are more akin to pillars than puzzle pieces. A weak link causes the entire structure to fall. You must provide your body with the right nutrients in order for it to adapt to your workout. You also need to workout properly if you want to increase your strength and muscular mass.

Your attempts to build muscle through strength training will be ineffective if you keep consuming a lot of calories that are devoid of nutrients and lack the proper ratio of macronutrients.

nutrients, both micro and macro

Minerals and vitamins make up micronutrients. These vitamins and minerals are necessary for our bodies to be healthy. They support the control of the heartbeat, metabolism, and bone density. Proteins, carbs, and fats make up macronutrients in contrast. For optimum performance, our bodies need a balance of macro- and micronutrients.

Proteins

Proteins are well known for enhancing strength and muscle growth. Our testosterone levels drop as we age, and our muscular mass follows suit. As a result, fat can replace muscle cells, causing unwanted weight gain or changes in body structure as well as weak muscles. You will need to consume more proteins if you want to gain muscle growth.

Even healthy seniors need more protein than they did when they were younger to help preserve muscle mass as we age because our metabolism slows down. As a result, it is advised that you eat 1.2–1.7 grams of protein per kilogram of your target body weight or 0.5–0.8 grams per pound of your target body weight each day.

Proteins are abundant in foods like tofu, fish, eggs, lean meat, beans, and legumes.

Choose complex carbohydrates when it comes to consuming carbohydrates. Avoid simple carbs, which are high in empty calories and include refined grains and added sugars, at all costs if you want to stay healthy. Oatmeal, whole grains, legumes (beans and lentils), sesame seeds, and other foods include complex carbohydrates.

Fat

Dietary fat is crucial because it fuels the body, aids in nutrient absorption, and supports the health of the neurological system. Both saturated and unsaturated fats are available to us. The distinction between the two is that unsaturated fats, which are thought to be the healthiest, are liquid at room temperature whereas saturated fats are solid.

Some unsaturated fatty acids are considered necessary nutrients, meaning that since our bodies can't produce them, we must obtain them through food. However, some foods, such as proteins from meat and poultry, may include unsaturated fats; as a result, it is essential to be selective when choosing them and remove any visible fat.

Your risk of stroke and cardiovascular disorders may be reduced if you choose unsaturated fats over saturated ones. You can eat healthy fats by eating nuts like cashew and almond or avocado. These fats are unsaturated. Conversely, meals high in saturated fats such shortening and fatty meats should be avoided.

Nutrition before and after exercise

It is crucial that you pay close attention to your pre- and post-workout nutrition. The foods you eat before and after exercising should be carefully chosen to balance your blood sugar levels, promote correct and quick recovery, and improve performance. As a result, it's crucial to think about eating a healthy food that will complement your exercise routine.

Exercise Nutrition

Depending on your training objective, you need to fuel your body with the appropriate nutrients in the appropriate amounts before you begin your workout. This helps you perform at your best by ensuring that your body has the energy to support lifting during the workout.

Consume items that will provide you enough energy to complete your last exercise prior to working out. Proteins and carbohydrates should be included in the meal.

These macronutrients each have a distinct function. However, their intake ratio changes based on your workout objective and type. For instance, you should eat less food, less carbohydrates, and more proteins before doing out if your objective is to lose weight. Additionally, your pre-workout meal should have larger portions and more proteins and carbohydrates if your goal is to develop muscle growth.

Let's examine the functions that each of these macronutrients performs when ingested before to exercise:

Carbs

When you exercise, carbs provide your muscles with fuel. You need more carbohydrates to keep going as your activity intensity increases. Carbohydrates aid in weight management and supply the energy required to carry out workout. Remember that during exercise, your muscles are fuelled by the glucose found in carbohydrates. This is why including "healthy" carbs in your pre-workout meal is crucial.

A "healthy" carb to eat before working out includes foods like bananas, oats, and whole grains. You should eat 0.25 to 0.5 grams of carbohydrates per pound of body weight three to four hours before working out. But keep in mind that this number drops as you get closer to your workout. For instance, if you have to eat an hour before your workout, you just need 0.25 grams of carbohydrates per pound of body weight.

Proteins

Who is unaware that proteins help develop muscle? Proteins are widely known for helping our bodies heal and rebuild. Protein ingestion before a workout boosts muscle protein synthesis, according to numerous studies. Additionally, it improves the anabolic response, boosts muscular mass and strength, and enhances performance and muscle recovery.

Before working out, yogurt or protein shakes are the finest options. It is advised to eat 20 grams of protein before working out.

Do you have a question about when to eat before working out? Ideally, 1-3 hours prior to your workout, you should fuel your body with the nutrients listed above. However, it is suggested that you have a comprehensive meal with proteins, fats, and some carbs about 2-3 hours before your workout if you want to maximize your results.

If for whatever reason you are unable to obtain a full meal during this time, you can still obtain a reasonable lunch. A snack might also be beneficial. However, you should be aware that if you must eat just before exercising, the meal should be easy to digest and smaller in size.

The top things to eat before working out are listed below:

Low-fat milk and oatmeal

Banana and a variety of fruit

Brown rice, whole-grain bread, and eggs

sandwich, vegetables, and lean protein

Fresh fruit and Greek yogurt

Chicken breast, a protein shake, and whole-grain cereal

Afterwards Nutrition

Don't overlook your post-workout diet as you work on your pre-workout nutrition. Eating the correct foods before and after exercise is equally crucial. You must grasp how physical exercise affects your body in order to appreciate the significance of eating the proper foods in the appropriate quantities and ratios.

I'll explain what happens in a nutshell: Your muscles burn up their glycogen reserves while you workout to fuel your body. This causes your muscles' glycogen reserves to partially deplete. Additionally, keep in mind that your body needs glucose to carry out daily tasks. Your body must therefore rebuild, repair, and develop new muscle proteins and restore the glycogen stores after exercise.

You must thus eat things that will help you do that after working out. Your post-workout diet should therefore include a lot of proteins and a few carbs. Experts advise eating your post-workout meals 45 minutes or less after working out. But it's best to eat as soon as possible.

Your glycogen stores will be refilled, and eating a balanced diet that includes protein and some carbohydrates will promote muscle growth and repair after exercise. Additionally, studies show that consuming 2040 grams of protein after working out helps muscles recover more quickly. Lean meat makes for the greatest protein. Eggs are another excellent choice.

Additionally, it is advised that you eat 0.5–0.7 grams of carbohydrates per pound of body weight after your workout. Oatmeal, potatoes, brown rice, fruits (banana, pineapple, and berries), and chocolate are some of the healthiest sources of carbohydrates. If your main objective is to lose extra weight, you can forgo the carbs after your workout and have a total of roughly 40 grams of protein.

Following an exercise, you might eat some of the following meals:

roasted veggies and grilled chicken

Yogurt with berries and little fat

cereals with fruits and nuts, wheat flakes, and oatmeal

fish and sweet potatoes

omelet with eggs and whole-wheat bread

with green beans in a burrito

mixed greens and chicken salad

With tofu and mushrooms

beef tenderloin served with brown rice

It is advisable to exercise in between meals or before your next one if you eat enough of each macronutrient at breakfast, lunch, and dinner. Additionally, if the interval between your activity and meals is too long, you might think about consuming supplements or snacks that are high in proteins and carbs.

Supplements

Just try your best to get all the nutrients you need from your diet when it comes to fitness. The importance of supplements is not as great as many believe. In actuality, you can attain your fitness goals without using supplements. The ideal ones, though, might hasten your success. Valid scientific research has demonstrated that several supplements can increase muscle growth and fat loss, increase performance and muscle recovery, and enhance general health. You can think about incorporating a few vitamins into your workout routine as a result.

For example, creatine, beta-alanine, and citrulline have all been shown to facilitate a faster increase in muscle growth and strength. Yohimbine and synephrine may also aid in fat burning, according to research. On the other hand, fish oil and vitamin D enhance your health and happiness.

It would require another book if I decided to dissect everything you see on the shelves of your neighborhood supplement retailer. In order to achieve your health and fitness goals, I'm just going to concentrate on a few supplement categories: fish oil, vitamin D, protein powder, fat burner, and muscle builder.

You may dramatically and positively impact your health by using these five different sorts of supplements. With the help of these supplements, you can increase your strength and muscle mass, reduce fat, strengthen your immune system, enhance your general health, and do even more. Let's examine each of them more closely.

one. Fish oil

Fish oil is exactly what it sounds like—fish oil. Popular options include sardines and salmon. Omega-3 fatty acids, which are crucial for developing muscle, are abundant in fish oil. These vital fatty acids are also necessary for our bodies to avoid sickness.

According to research, our diet barely contains about a tenth of these fatty acids on average. Because of this, supplementing may be a wise decision. Omega-3 fatty acid intake has been demonstrated to:

Reduced stress, anxiety, and depression

Reduce joint and muscle discomfort

keep you from gaining too much weight

Boost excess fat loss Boost rapid muscular growth

Boost mental performance.

2. Calcium

For strong bones, vitamin D is necessary. It can fend off osteoporosis and aid calcium absorption in the bones. It also has a significant impact on physiological processes like metabolism, immune system performance, and cell division and growth. This suggests that a lack of vitamin D can cause major issues for your body.

Vitamin D can be obtained by food, sunlight, or supplements. Few foods, including cow liver, cheese, and egg yolk, naturally contain vitamin D, but the amounts are quite modest. The majority of individuals acquire their vitamins from sunlight, but as we age, our bodies become less able to turn sunlight into vitamin D. As a result, taking supplements is the simplest and most trustworthy way to increase your body's vitamin D levels.

Speaking of other vitamin supplements, the majority of individuals can obtain all the vitamins and minerals they require by eating a healthy, balanced diet, therefore they are generally not required to take them.

Fat Burner 3.

I don't have to mention this anymore. But I'll say it anyway: There isn't a pill or powder on the market that can make you stronger, healthier, or more attractive.

That is the unfortunate reality, believe it or not. I'll give it to you without charge.

There isn't a secure "fat-burning" substance strong enough to result in appreciable fat loss on its own. Anyone who makes the claim to offer you such goods is defrauding you. Spending hundreds of dollars a month on useless supplements to feed steroid-fueled bodybuilders is a waste.

Additionally, you shouldn't be shocked that the majority of bodybuilding and weight reduction products available are duds. Fortunately, there are a few supplements that can speed up your weight reduction progress—but only if you know how to properly fuel it with sensible dieting and exercise. One of the few dietary supplements that research has shown to be useful in this area is caffeine.

4. Bodybuilders

Some people become frustrated after spending a lot of money on muscle-building pills that don't produce the desired results. You should now be aware that the majority of the well-known products on the market that promote muscle building actually accomplish nothing. Fortunately, there are a few that have been shown by research to be successful. One of the very few supplements you can utilize to promote muscle growth is creatine.

5. Powdered protein

If you believe you struggle to consume enough proteins in your diet for one reason or another, you might want to consider investing in a high-quality protein powder (for example, you could be allergic to most of them). On the market, a variety of protein powders are available, including vegan-friendly varieties. They exist to guarantee that you are consuming enough protein to successfully create muscles. All you need to do is stir in a scoop to your preferred beverage to get started. You can also benefit from consuming 20 grams of whey protein before or after working out.

Hydration

The human body needs water to function properly. Your body is composed of roughly 70% water. The pace at which we lose water from our bodies increases with exercise. We frequently lose a significant amount of water and electrolytes through sweating during and after exercise.

In order to attain your fitness goals, it is crucial that you include a healthy hydration strategy in your training regimen.

Not only is staying adequately hydrated important during exercise, but it's also important in general. "Water is life," they say. Dehydration from insufficient fluid intake might interfere with your body's normal functions. Electrolytes and bodily fluids are lost when one is dehydrated. Without these vital components, your body cannot function properly.

Exercise performance can suffer if you're dehydrated since it makes you feel too tired and lethargic to work out. It also causes headaches and cramping in the muscles. Additionally, working out while dehydrated puts your muscular strength and endurance at danger.

The necessity of bodily hydration

It enhances the effectiveness of your workouts. Dehydration can cause abnormal body temperatures, increased weariness, cramping in the muscles, and decreased motivation. All of them increase the perceived physical and mental difficulty of exercise. It is simpler to exercise when you drink enough water and other fluids to prevent dehydration.

Water aids in quicker digestion by accelerating the breakdown of food and the absorption of nutrients ingested before and after exercise.

Important minerals and electrolytes that we lose through sweating during exercise can be found in abundance in water and other fluids.

In order for joints to go through their full range of motion during exercise, they need to be lubricated. Water serves as a shock absorber as well.

Water aids in weight loss as well. A glass of water before a meal has been shown in numerous studies to reduce hunger and increase metabolism, which helps with weight loss.

Maintaining proper hydration promotes healthy skin.

I'll remind you that you should aim to consume 8 glasses, or 2 liters, of water each day.

Main Points

It's not necessary to deprive yourself of your favorite foods and consume bland dishes when dieting properly. Eating the meals you enjoy while staying in shape is possible.

The dietary requirements of various people vary depending on their body types, ages, and fitness objectives.

Use what you already have as a starting point for your diet plan.

Pre-workout meals should be consumed two to three hours before exercising.

Within 45 minutes of your workout, eat your post-workout meal. Better would be sooner.

If you consume a healthy diet, you won't require supplements. Try as much as possible to receive all your nutrients from a whole food diet.

You cannot become healthy, stronger, or attractive by taking a pill or powder.

(For more detail on nutrition, see my books "Healthy Eating for Men" or "MACRO Diet Cookbook").

Chapter 5

Maintaining Consistency

"If done consistently, a simple daily task will outweigh a spasmodic Hercules' labors."

Tony Trollope

Always maintain consistency. Success depends on being consistent. Similar to how you must continually work at anything else in your life if you want to succeed, so too must your fitness objective be accomplished. Any fitness goal, whether it be weight loss, growing muscular mass and strength, or any other particular objective, must be consistently pursued to be successful. To get the most out of your activities, you must put forth consistent effort and be dedicated to your training regimen.

Typically, muscle growth is a progressive process that happens over time and is slow and constant. Your stamina won't develop and your workouts won't become more effective and efficient until you maintain consistency. If you know in the back of your mind that you don't require extensive breaks from your workouts, don't use that as an excuse.

The first step to achieving consistency is having a straightforward workout schedule, which we already have in chapter 6. Guess what, then? You have already made some progress toward achieving consistency. A smart workout schedule should keep you on track and correspond to your fitness objectives.

Every workout has a well-defined plan so that you won't have to worry as much about the exercises you need to complete or what you need to accomplish in your next workout.

A good fitness plan should also focus on workouts that work out your full body muscles. That's what chapter 6 of my book proposes to do. However, it's crucial to understand that even if you have the most effective and ideal workout plan in place, it won't help you in the slightest if you aren't consistent and follow it.

Your body undergoes a lot of changes while you workout. Your body goes through specific processes and releases substances (hormones) that cause your body to alter in various ways. Your body changes and gets more robust and efficient as you exercise because more reactions and secretions are produced.

This means that if you exercise consistently, your body will adjust to the changes, enabling you to get stronger and exercise more effectively.

Your muscles become harmed from training when you constantly undertake demanding exercises. Your muscle cells' organelles are disrupted as a result, and the satellite cells are then activated. The hormones in your body then trigger the satellite cells, increasing the size of your muscle fibers.

We all want to have a body that is powerful, healthy, and appealing. But you must realize that in order to accomplish even one of these objectives, if not all of them, you must accept consistency. Making exercise a habit will help you stay committed to it. The exercises grow more natural the more often you do them.

Initially, things could appear difficult. You could even feel like giving up. But refrain. The rest will fall into place if you only keep in mind that consistency is the key to unlocking success in your training goals. That's all, after your body adjusts. In actuality, you won't ever want to skip a workout. However, you must practice consistency before coming here. The more you exercise, the more accustomed your body will acquire to it, and the more it will resemble a pastime, if not a habit.

How to Maintain Consistency

Prepare for challenges. Consider all the scenarios where you might need to take longer pauses from exercising and make plans for them. Take initiative. Everyday obstacles that we all run against can occasionally cause us to stumble or fall. You are more equipped to proceed both physically and psychologically if you have a plan on how to overcome these challenges. If you occasionally need to attend activities after work, you might plan your calendar such that it is less hectic. Additionally, you must account for inclement weather and other timing constraints.

Use recollections. It is quite simple to forget to do new things until they become habits when you first start doing them because they are not a part of your regular routine. You can overlook the necessity to exercise on a specific day. You might even forget occasionally that you're following an exercise regimen. Set reminders on your phone, calendar, watch, or even smart assistants to make sure you don't forget to exercise. You can also print your exercise schedule and adhere it to a surface like your desk, refrigerator, or mirror.

Avoid thinking anything bad. Every achievement begins in the mind. You are what you believe you are. Most of us let our thoughts undermine our intentions and objectives. You'll understand what I'm talking about if you're familiar with the proverb "we are our worst enemy." You're less likely to exercise consistently if you're constantly thinking "I can't," "I am not," and other negative statements.

Be devoted. Being committed entails carrying through an action even when it is not convenient or something you don't feel like doing. Another essential factor for success is commitment. You must be dedicated if you want to achieve in anything. As a result, you must commit to working out for at least 30 days if you want to establish consistency in your workouts. Exercise can help you stay committed if you do it once, twice, or three times per week for a month. Are you perplexed as to why a month? According to research, it takes an average person 24 days of doing something repeatedly to form a habit.

Decide on a goal. Focus more on creating short-term objectives. Some long-term objectives could seem impossible to achieve and be unreasonable. Make sure your objective is SMART (Specific - Measurable - Achievable - Relevant - Time-limited) before you put it in writing. Make a connection with it so that it has a deep meaning in your life. Go above and beyond to provide the motivations for having such a goal, as well as the anticipated rewards of reaching the goal. To acquire more muscle mass and vitality, take care of yourself, and play with your kids, for instance, instead of setting a goal like "exercise frequently," plan to do so 2-3 days a week for the following 18 weeks.

Maintain a good exercise schedule. One of the simplest ways to fail when starting a fitness quest is without a set exercise schedule. Probably familiar with the adage "What gets scheduled, gets done" It is simpler to state that you will workout; however, actually doing it is another matter. When you arrange your workout on your calendar or planner, it becomes more genuine.

Additionally, it helps you be more responsible, remain on schedule, and prioritize exercise.

Start modest as you progress progressively. Do not jump right into adding more sets and reps and lifting bigger weights. Move slowly. Most people who stop working out always begin at a pace they can't keep up for very long. Start light and gradually increase the intensity of your workout, sets/reps, and weight as you gain strength.

Be tolerant. Rome "wasn't constructed in a day," as you are well aware. Muscles do not grow overnight. Most individuals assume that results will always be visible straight immediately. Such goals are unattainable. If you find that you're not entirely following your exercise plan, you must also have patience with yourself. You must be aware that developing a new habit can take some time. Be patient and have faith in the process. Everything will come into focus.

Look for responsibility. When others are watching, people are more inclined to adhere to their fitness schedule religiously. Find an accountability partner so that you can truly commit to making the adjustments. This might be your partner, a close friend, or even a relative. Nobody wants to let down their loved one or their workout partner. Select a partner with whom you can commit to a similar exercise regimen as your accountability buddy.

Track your development. Weekly evaluations of your development will reveal your accomplishments. Record any advancements you made. When you realize what you have accomplished, it inspires you to work out more and do better at the things you believe you need to work on.

Make working out pleasurable. Find several ways to add enjoyment to your training. You may associate it with a fun activity, like playing a game, do it outside with friends, or treat yourself to support your regular effort.

For you to have a physique that is healthier, stronger, fitter, and leaner, you must incorporate exercise into your daily life. When carefully considered, the aforementioned advice will assist you in maintaining consistency in your exercise routine and achieving lasting transformation.

Exercise Stagnation

Our bodies typically experience periods of stagnation. When your workout program is properly followed but you don't notice any change or positive outcomes, you are said to be in workout stagnation. Stagnation typically happens when your muscles become accustomed to a certain workout schedule and the same stimulation you give them every day. As a result, you do your workouts less effectively, your muscles stop expanding, and your body stops tracking your progress toward gaining muscle.

Stasis during a workout is usual and expected. Each person experiences it. If you haven't already, you will eventually get there as you exercise. You must alter your workout's plan and approach when it becomes stagnant. What you should do is as follows:

up your reps and sets. For instance, if you've been performing 3 sets of 6 repetitions, up the number of sets to 4 or use lighter weight for 10 repetitions. As you advance and your body adjusts, it is advised to switch up your reps and sets.

Before you begin exercising, warm up. Before you start your workout, stimulate your muscles by doing some warm-up activities like running in place.

Adapt your exercise program. Use different exercises from chapter 4 to redefine and adapt your existing training regimen. Here, all we're attempting to do is work out our muscles from various angles. Your body will now have fresh stimulus for building muscle.

Make a nutrition plan to support your exercise regimen. Make sure your nutrition plan helps your body get the nutrients and energy it needs before and after a workout.

Reduce the repetition rate. Your muscles can experience greater time under stress as a result, allowing them to move through their whole range of motion.

Try to do your exercises in less time than you anticipated. Your muscles can expand by being exposed to new stimuli by performing more exercises in less time.

Strike a balance between intensity and volume. Do not ever ignore your body. Reduce the number of sessions you complete each week if your workout intensity is high, and raise the number of sessions if it is low.

Your body responds by generating new muscles to handle the circumstances at hand when you subject your muscles to a given training intensity. But keep in mind that these forces are continually and repeatedly stressed, thus your body must continue to build new muscles. In order to assist your muscles develop new strength to handle the stress, you must be consistent with your workouts.

When you establish consistency, it is incredibly satisfying. On the other side, it is really irritating when you don't succeed because it means you also didn't fulfill your goal.

You already know that if you want to obtain your desired body shape or any other training objective, you must remain dedicated to your workouts.

It's also crucial to realize that the majority of people constantly give up when faced with consistency problems, and you can be one of them. But don't make that decision. You won't have the opportunity to meet your targeted fitness goal. Just give yourself some grace.

Remember that developing consistency is a patience-based talent. Simply persevere through all of the difficulties that arise while working out, and consistency will come.

Key Takeaways Your best tool in the fight to meet your strength training objectives is consistency. Maintain consistency with your diet, recovery, and exercise routines.

Chapter 6

FAQs

"Try being weak if you think lifting is risky. Being fragile is risky.

B. Contreras

Q1: I've never exercised before; is it too late to start now?

Never let it be too late. Even if you've never worked out, you can start right away and enjoy the same advantages as those who strength train when they're younger. According to experts, seniors who have led sedentary lifestyles can begin a regular exercise routine at any age.

I'm not suggesting that you start exercising when you're 80. Keep in mind that if you wait that long, you risk hurting yourself. Your whole muscular mass will be lost. Maintaining the health of your bones and muscles through strength training. Additionally, studies indicate that starting an exercise program later in life can still help you reduce your chance of developing age-related health issues.

I am not overweight; thus, do I really need to exercise?

Even if you are not overweight, you could still be weak or have other health conditions that affect your bones. A healthy and fit body is not necessarily one that is slim. I'm saying that regular exercise is necessary for maintaining excellent health and lowering health risks. even if your doctor says your weight is a healthy amount. Most 'age-related' health issues are more likely to occur if you lead a sedentary lifestyle. Thus, frequent exercise is important. whether or not you are overweight.

Q3: I have a number of health issues. Is it safe to exercise?

It is advisable to speak with your doctor before beginning any exercise regimen. Tell him/her about your condition and inquire about any special safety measures you should take as well as the exercises that are appropriate for you.

According to research, regular exercise can reduce the risk of developing chronic diseases and hasten the healing process after serious illnesses like heart attack, stroke, joint replacement surgery, and many others. Due of this, many medical professionals might advise exercise even in the wake of a catastrophic accident or illness.

Exercise also protects against osteoporosis, keeps your body flexible, and stabilizes your joints, reducing your risk of injury. Exercise is safe and beneficial even if you have medical concerns; in fact, it will help you manage those conditions, which is the short answer to this question.

Is exercise really necessary for me at this age?

You are never too old. Age is not a barrier to fitness. You may strength train at any age and yet enjoy all of its advantages. Being physically inactive is really riskier and has been shown to speed up aging. Compared to non-exercisers, people who exercise regularly have a twofold lower risk of developing chronic illnesses.

Compared to when you were younger, you now require more regular exercise. Yes. Your body was capable of taking care of itself back then. But as time goes on, your metabolism slows down, you lose muscle mass year after year, and fat now tends to build up so quickly. Because of their fragility, your bones are more prone to breaking. This calls for action on your part. Work hard now to develop the muscle and arteries of a 20-year-old. All of those signs of aging can be reversed with a solid exercise regimen.

Q5. How soon after you stop exercising do you start losing muscle?

Once you begin your strength training program, you might be concerned that taking a break would cause you to lose the strength and muscle mass that you have worked so hard to build. In fact, taking a few days off from exercise can help you reach your fitness objectives by giving your muscles time to heal. The issue arises, though, when we take excessively long rests.

According to some research, if you go too long between workouts, you may begin to lose muscle as soon as one week and as much as 2 pounds if you are completely immobile. And according to another study, even when you're not bedridden, your muscle mass might shrink by roughly 11% after ten days of inactivity.

It's crucial to understand that actual muscle atrophy often occurs at times of injury or when you entirely stop utilizing your muscles for a prolonged length of time before you freak out and start regretting every vacation or week off you've ever had. You can rest for roughly three weeks without experiencing a significant loss in muscular strength.

However, a variety of factors, such as the following, affect how rapidly you lose muscle mass after you stop exercising.

how frequently and for how long you've been working out. The muscles you have are a result of how long you've been exercising. You will have more muscles if you consistently lift weights over a longer period of time. This puts you in a better position even if you choose to pause your program or are forced to do so. Even if you remain inactive for a while, you will still have a baseline of muscle that others won't because you will be fit with developed muscles.

the diet. In particular, we require enough protein to develop and sustain muscular mass. People who don't get enough protein don't have enough amino acids to keep up with the daily breakdown and repair of bodily cells. Your body eventually extracts the amino acids from your muscles and uses them to maintain the health of your other cells and tissues. Muscle loss is the effect of this. So even if you aren't training, it is crucial to make sure you are getting enough protein.

Age. It is more difficult to gain and maintain muscle mass as we age due to a number of factors. One of them is the alteration in the coordination of our nerve systems. We typically lose motor neurons as we age. Motor neurons help muscles contract more forcefully by directing spinal cord impulses to the muscles. Therefore, it becomes challenging to recruit new muscle fibers if you lose them. Strength training therefore aids in the reversal of these as well as many other age-related alterations. However, the advantages progressively fade if you quit exercising.

Sex. Males have a little advantage over females when it comes to muscle loss because they naturally produce testosterone, which is anabolic to the growth and maintenance of muscle tissue.

How do I choose the proper weight for a kettlebell?

You are free to perform a test to see if you can support the weight of the kettlebell you intend to use during your workout. Start by trying to perform many reps of the kettlebell military press in the store to choose a good weight. That is the appropriate weight for you to manage. Even though you'll need the lightest weight for this exercise, you can also use it for the other exercises. Keep in mind that it is best to learn the motions slowly than to risk hurting yourself.

Q7: Can testosterone replacement therapy (TRT) increase the effectiveness of my workouts?

Yes. In reality, the majority of the well-built males I have met admit that TRT is their secret. Your testosterone hormone levels start to fall at the age of 30, and they steadily rise as you become older (Mayo Clinic, 2020). In order to get the most out of your weightlifting routines, you might need to increase your testosterone if you find that it is excessively low.

However, I favor natural ways to increase your testosterone levels over TRT. Everyone is aware that doing things naturally has very few, if any, negative side effects. According to research, TRT may result in a decrease in sperm count, an increased risk of blood clots and heart attacks, the encouragement of noncancerous prostate growth, larger breasts, shrinkage of the testicles, and other side effects. You can go TRT until you are prepared for all of this.

Consuming vitamins and supplements like zinc, vitamin B, and vitamin D is one of the greatest strategies to maintain or raise your testosterone levels. Other methods include eating right, exercising, and getting enough sleep (7 to 10 hours).

CAN YOU PLEASE DO ME A FAVOR?

Your reading of Strength Training Over 40 is appreciated. I sincerely hope you put what you've discovered to use to look, feel, and live better than you ever have.

I have a small favor to ask.

Would you mind taking a moment to review this book on Amazon? I read every review, and I appreciate sincere criticism. Real compensation for my work comes from knowing that I am assisting others.

>> Give Amazon US a brief review by clicking here. Please consider leaving a brief review on Amazon UK. I appreciate your time and look forward to hearing from you.

Conclusion

All advancement occurs outside of one's comfort zone, according to Michael John Bobak.

It is impossible to overstate the many advantages of strength training. regardless of age. Never let it be too late. You must be aware that if we continue to be physically inactive beyond the age of 30, the much-discussed loss of muscle mass gets worse.

You can increase your muscle mass, manage chronic conditions, strengthen your bones, and do a lot more with strength training. This book offers all you need if you want to maintain your health, strength, and physical fitness.

If you've been reading along, you should know at this point that strength training is the best option if you want to build a strong, healthy, and fit body. If you're new to strength training, it could be frightening to make this kind of commitment because it pushes you outside of your cozy comfort zone. But if you want to accomplish this priceless aim, that is your only option. You'll succeed if you only approach it with the correct attitude!

Main Points

Your strength training needs the appropriate kind of drive. Find out why you exercise. You will be able to do whatever is necessary to accomplish them if you do this. Making time for training may seem like an impossible chore, but with careful planning, you will have enough of it.

Start out slowly and steadily as you train. Set sensible objectives and continue to put in great effort to achieve them. Keep in mind that if you don't have a goal or destination in mind, you are more likely to fail. Imagine one. Be patient while you start your training as well. The process of getting a strong, healthy, and fit body also takes time. A quality wine takes years to age in a bottle. Therefore, be patient!

Exercise doesn't require a lot of equipment. There is no need for pricey or specialized gym equipment to perform strength training. Nevertheless, it is a good idea to spend money on a few pieces of gear. Equipment for weightlifting that is reasonably priced and effective is available.

Equipment that costs a lot of money is not necessary. You have everything you need to reap great benefits from your training regimen without breaking the bank with only one kettlebell. You'll discover that it's worthwhile, and you won't look back. Although you can still use your body weight to attain your strength training goals, I think using free weights, especially a kettlebell, is the best choice.

Plan your workouts. Whoever doesn't plan, plans to fail. I have created a fitness schedule that is customized for YOU. Make sure to follow this program for at least four weeks if you want to experience the full benefits of strength training. You'll be able to maintain your route and workout efficiently. Be consistent and keep in mind that you should increase the weight, reps, or sets you use to gradually overload your muscles.

Follow a healthy diet. Never undervalue the role that nutrition plays in helping you reach your fitness objectives. Remember that the success or failure of any strength training program will depend on your diet. Take care with the food you eat. This does not entail depriving yourself of your favorite dishes and eating only bland fare. You can eat the meals you enjoy and still stay in shape.

You must provide your body the nutrients it needs first since they are good. Additionally, you can take supplements if you can't get enough of them from your diet. However, I strongly advise people to make every effort to obtain all of their nutrients through whole foods rather than supplements. Processed foods are among the items you should avoid, on the other hand. Sugary and processed foods should be avoided since they will impair your health.

Protein intake recommendations range from 1.2 to 1.7 grams per kilogram of target body weight or 0.5 to 0.8 grams per pound of target body weight per day.

You should eat 20 to 40 grams of protein both before and after your workout.

Supersets are the most efficient approach to complete your exercises and maximize your workout time.

To gain the advantages of both muscle and strength building, you must complete 3 sets of 6–12 repetitions.

Additionally, you must train 1-3 days per week, with days off in between.

Make sure to exercise safely. Keep in mind that maintaining fitness, muscle mass, and strength is the main objective here, along with maintaining good health and avoiding injuries. Make sure to workout correctly. Avoid pressing too hard too quickly. Start small and rise through the ranks. When performing the motions, have good form. Your security is crucial. Limit your muscular use. Give them time to heal.

Be dependable. Remember that your best tool for getting the body you want is consistency.

Finally, you must maintain appropriate hydration. To avoid being dehydrated when exercising, drink plenty of water before, during, and after. Ideally, you should consume 8 glasses, or 2 liters, of water each day. So make sure you consume 2 liters or more of water each day.

The most surefire way to reach your fitness objectives is through strength training in conjunction with healthy eating, rest, and water.

You will love the benefits if you are consistent and make sure you exercise safely.

You have all you need now, so start looking for that strong, fit, and healthy body. If you don't put more effort into putting what you've learned in this book into practice, it will all be for nothing and have no impact on how you look or live. Having pleasure and being content while doing what you love is the most essential thing in anyone's life. Strength training ought to be one of those things, as it is for me.

Printed by BoD˝in Norderstedt, Germany